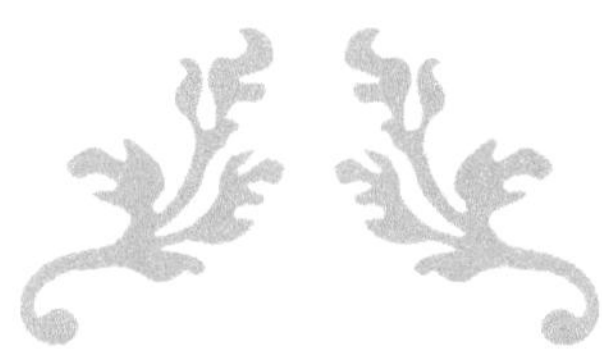

FAITH. HOPE. CURE. GASTROPARESIS

Cookbook

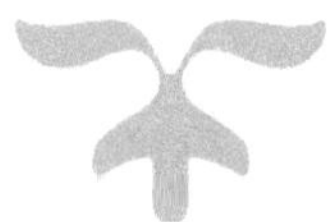

By: Melissa Gordon

Table of Contents

<u>*Chapter 1*</u>

Hi everyone, nice to meet you, my name is Missy, and I'm a gastroparesis warrior, just like you.

I know what you're thinking; well at least I hope I do. It's difficult to have this terrible disease, and going through it as well. It's truly a pain in the butt. But don't be discouraged because I've worked really hard with myself to make sure I don't suffer too much with this gastroparesis. I eat a lot of soups, some white beans and rice, and pizza only if I make it myself. Basically, I cook a lot of my own foods, and my family helps me out as well. And of course, I can't forget to mention the positive encouragement I receive from my wonderful audience with whom I will now share my wonderful cooking and meals.

I really hope you guys will enjoy the meals as much as I love making them. And I pray it will and hope it will help you as well, and if it doesn't then, talk to your doctor about what will work for you. I can only help you so much because you've also got to do what it takes to help your amazing self.

You're also probably wondering why I'm about to give you a vocabulary lesson on our stomach problem. Well, I don't know if you know what gastroparesis is or not, so I hope you don't mind if I tell you a little bit about what it is, based off what I know about it.

<u>Definition of Gastroparesis</u>:

It's a condition that affects the normal muscle movements of the stomach.

Very common (More than 3 million cases per year in the US)

Diagnosis often requires a lab test or imaging

No known cure, treatments available

Can be lifelong

Gastroparesis is said to be caused by damaged nerves of the stomach. The symptoms include constant nausea and vomiting. The treatment includes medication and diet.

<u>Chapter 2</u>

Symptoms:

- Nausea

- Vomiting, especially vomiting undigested food a few hours after eating

- Feeling of fullness even after eating very little

- Acid reflux or heartburn

- Abdominal pain and/or bloating

- Changes in blood sugar levels

- Lack of appetite and malnutrition

- Weight loss

Gastroparesis Starving for a Cure by: Melissa Gordon

Treatments:

There is no cure for gastroparesis. Treatments aim at reducing or managing symptoms, by treating the underlying conditions.

Self-Care:

- Maintain adequate nutrition

- Consume easier to digest foods

- Eat well- cooked fruits and vegetables

These are some of the things that I learned by researching the illness myself and what my doctor has helped me understand. My special amazing doctor teaches me a lot of things about gastroparesis, and I helped her as well. I'm so grateful to have my awesome doctor, and I know the knowledge she gave me will help you too.

Fortunately, I know my doctor personally, she's first and foremost an amazing doctor to me. Secondly, she's a very caring and loving person who wants to help anyone who comes to see her. So, I recommend that you find a doctor who is knowledgeable and friendly just like my doctor.

Personal Quote: *Always believe in yourself even though, you feel like giving up sometimes. Keep on fighting no matter what and keep on moving forward. Because good things are coming your way no matter what. Keep on praying wonderful things.*

Ok, so now that we have gotten all the heavy things I wanted to say out of the way, here comes the fun part. I do this all for me; I eat the right foods and walk a lot to try and stay as healthy as possible. I will be honest with you, I do have some ups and downs just like you do, but I push myself to make it through each day and pray a whole lot. Each day I say to myself, **"I can do it! I believe in myself!"**

And if I can do it, so can you. So, let's hear you say, I can do it! And now you can move forward into your amazing life. So now here are some of my cooking recipes which I hope you will all enjoy.

Chapter 3

If you have gastroparesis like me, I recommend that you limit the intake of certain foods. Here is a list of some of the foods that I avoid.

"Foods to Avoid"

- No steak, no red meat of any kind
- No ground beef, no burgers made with beef
- No milk (milk hurts your already sore tummy)
- No pizza with red sauce
- No sodas

- No salads

- No pasta

- No coffee

- No peanuts (of any kind)

- No hard fruit (like apples, applesauce ok)

- No ham

- No pork of any kind (pork is red meat)

And there are so many more foods, but ask your doctor about your food restriction list as well, so that you know what you can't eat. I only named a few that I avoid for myself based on what I do at home.

"Foods You Can Eat"

- Cane fruits

- Baked chicken of any kind

- Cheese of any kind

- Potatoes of any kind

- Oatmeal

- Cream of wheat

- Eggs whites

And a whole lot of soups! chicken broth is my number one go to thing! Creamy white soups are the best. Remember, no red soups all. Tomato based soups are bad for you.

So far so good right? Now I will list a few meals we can eat and a few meals to avoid. But remember, if this doesn't help you, can always ask your doctor for help on this as well.

Start off by making sure you eat lots of peanut butter, the natural kind, and strawberry jelly that's sugar-free with a glass of dairy-free milk. That will make sure you are completely full. Enjoy!!

Now, where are those awesome cooking skills that I inherited from my family?

"Recipes"

Chapter 4

Basic Chicken Broth Soup

(serves 2-3 people)

Ingredients:

- 1 tablespoon of powdered chicken broth

- 5 cups of water total

- 1 cup of baked chicken (already cooked, diced or ripped into pieces)

- 2 carrots (diced)

- 1 potato – (cook one whole potato then dice)

- 1 stalk of celery (diced)

- garlic powder and onion powder to taste (1 tsp to start)

You'll need to gather the following materials to begin cooking. Get a large stock pot and put it on the stove, turn on the temperature dial to around 6 or 7 (medium high) and let the pot get warmed up. Then, take a measuring cup and pour a tablespoon of powered chicken broth into a one cup measuring cup. Add some water to the cup with granules and blend until all chicken granules have dissolved. Add mixture to your pot.

To ensure that the soup is not too salty, add four additional cups of water. Then add carrots, chicken and potatoes to the pot and cook it all together.

Then add the onion and garlic powder to taste. You can add whatever other seasonings you wish to add at this time. Some ideas include: oregano, cilantro, basil and turmeric, all of these will add flavor and be easy to digest. This is what I do with my meals at home. Have fun experimenting with your awesome seasonings for this ridiculously easy and amazing soup I make here at home.

And if you keep eating soup like this the way that I do; I know for a fact you will lose weight and look good too. And as an additional benefit you'll be helping your fabulous stomach as well.

Chapter 5

I know going through this pain daily may be hard to do, but you can survive this if you just believe in yourself.

More Recipes and Meal Ideas by Yours Truly

I highly recommend the combination of white beans and jasmine rice. Both of these items can be purchased in easy to prepare forms so that all you have to do is heat them up. If you purchase canned beans you should rinse them to reduce flatulence. It doesn't bother me at all when I eat them. But you really need to stay away from all the other beans. If you can eat them with no issues then that's great, but if you can't, then I say stay away from them for good.

So, what else do I like to eat besides soups? Well, here are my few of my favorites.

<u>Baked Potato and Grilled Chicken</u>

I cook my chicken (whatever chicken you have on hand) on the grill outside or on an indoor grill and I add some seasonings to it. Feel free to experiment with your seasonings like you did with the chicken soup. Ginger can help with nausea. Chicken must cook to an internal temperature of 165 degrees F in order to ensure that it will be completely done. Remember to keep an eye on your chicken so that it won't burn.

Now for the baked potato, you can cook it however you like really, some microwaves even have a baked potato button. What I do is to peel off the skin of the potato, wash it off in the sink and then cut it into small pieces. Once the pieces are boiled in water I can eat them as they are or make mash potatoes which is easier. Then you can add butter and light sour cream. Serve this with your grilled chicken and there you go, you have an easy to digest meal.

I recommend that you only eat half portions of your meal so that you won't get sick. And if you are having any problems at all, talk to your doctor about your situation.

Now we can move onto the fun part of my meal plan which is making yummy desserts. But only proceed if your digestion can handle them. If not, I'm very sorry and I wish you all the best in your heath. But, this is something I like to do to treat myself.

The dessert ideas I include are sugar-free foods or drinks. I hope you like these ideas and they will help you as well, so that you can have them just like me.

<u>Chapter 6</u>

I also make cakes and pies, as well. I try to do only sugar-free foods because those are the best ones. I hope you understand why I let myself have the desserts. I don't really cook that many desserts but when I do, they are super yummy in your tummy. You will love and enjoy them so much.

For the first recipe that I like to make often, I use a Red Velvet cake mix from a box. Then I add marshmallows, chocolate chips or light whipped cream.

Also, to make easy s'mores, put a gram cracker on a plate (break it in half,) then place the marshmallow on top. Cook it in the microwave just a few seconds until marshmallow melts down some. Then take it out of the microwave, and put the chocolate bar on top and the remaining gram cracker half on top- now you have your s'mores sandwich.

Creamy Peanut Butter Hot Chocolate Drink

Ingredients:

- 1 tablespoon chocolate protein powder or hot chocolate mix
- 1 tablespoon peanut butter protein powder
- 1 ½ teaspoon honey
- ½ cup of milk

Add all of these into a saucepan and boil together. It will be a wonderful drink to make and you'll love it so much.

<u>Apple Pie in A Bowl</u>

Ingredients:

- apple (1 or 2 cut up)
- butter 1 teaspoon
- bowl
- cinnamon seasoning

Cut up the apples, put them into a bowl then take the skin and seeds out and off. Add some butter to the bowl and add cinnamon.

Heat the mixture up in the microwave for 5 or 6 minutes, until done. And let stand for 1 minute and enjoy your apple pie.

Apple Pie Smoothie

Ingredients:

- 1 or 2 apples (cut up)
- 1 cup milk
- 1 tablespoon honey
- 1 tablespoon yogurt
- cinnamon powder (add as much as you like)

Put all the ingredients in a blender until smooth and drink. Enjoy this wonderful treat I make.

<u>*Chapter 7*</u>

Make sure you're getting lots of rest and the right amount of food in your tummy, not too much food, but not too little. And if you're on a liquid or restricted diet then, you might want to try some of the following foods:

- Jell-O (plain only)
- water
- bread (whole wheat only)
- milk (dairy free)
- yogurt (dairy free)
- plain broth soup from a can
- some plain crackers

When I have an upset tummy, I drink a lot of ginger ale sodas; this is called the ***Ginger Ale Sodas Diet***. This helps me out a whole lot, and it might help you as well. And I drink lots and lots of water too. These sodas will do the trick on you in a hurry, so if you are feeling nauseous then drink one of these, and it will help your tummy to feel better.

I can also say that there is another type of drink that has really help me out a lot as well. And I'm hoping they will work on you too. I get big packs of these drinks in many different flavors at Sam's Club, Smiths, and Walmart. And look for the Christmas edition of these drinks as well. These drinks are called

<u>Sparkling Ice Sodas</u>. And who knows, they may help you out as well.

I can also say whatever you do, stay away from the lemonade. That right there is bad for your poor tummy.

Chapter 8

I may not know that much about **"Gastroparesis"** but, I can tell you, this is what I do for self-care here at home. I really hope this will help you as well. And if it doesn't, then please talk to your doctor and get some help.

My Personal Quote: "You are not sick. You are trying to hang on and fight your gastroparesis, your sickness, like me. Now fight with Me!"

Not talking about your stomach problem, will only make it worse for you in the long run. So please, if this helps you and if you enjoy doing what I do, then go for it. And if this doesn't then, go get some help from your doctor. And if you want my advice then I say go see my amazing and special awesome doctor who wants to see you healthy and doing well.

I'm not saying my gastroparesis is cured or anything. No, that won't happen. But, if I keep telling my doctor what is wrong with me, and how I'm feeling and doing then I know what I'll do, and everything will be ok. And I will keep doing what I'm doing for myself as well.

And that's what keeps me eating right, losing weight, being positive and always praying that you and I will heal and get better one day soon enough.

Like I said before, never give up on yourself. And keep up the good work, because you are a winner, a fighter, an achiever and you can conquer this world.

I believe *in you* 100% and now you got to believe in *yourself*. And honey, you can put your mind to anything your heart believes in.

And I will pray and you do the same thing for myself as well.

Now let's ***cure our disease and conquer*** the world, the way we want it to happen.

Chapter 9
<u>Extra Soup Meals:</u>

<u>Potato Pasta Soup</u>

Another yummy thing I like to eat is potato soup with just a little bit of pasta.

Ingredients:

- 1 tablespoon chicken broth powder
- water

- 1 cup cooked sausage

- 1 cup diced celery

- 1 cup frozen corn

- 1 cup cooked potatoes

- 1 cup pasta

- 1 tablespoon flour

- seasonings (garlic, parsley, onion powder)

- milk

You'll make this soup the same way as the chicken soup but with some pasta. Put a pot onto the stove, bring your water to a boil, add a cup of noodles to the pot and the celery and boil them, until they are cooked and soft. (See recommended time on the box for noodle type.) Then add a tablespoon of chicken broth powder to a one cup measuring cup, fill it up water, whisk, then stir it into the pot. Then add sausage, potatoes, corn, carrots, chicken, some milk, and whisk a tablespoon flour into the pot as well. Cook until all vegetables are soft. And that's another amazing soup you will love as well. I know you will enjoy it very much.

Chicken Pot Pie Soup

Ingredients:

- chicken (1 cup)
- 1 tablespoon chicken broth powder
- 1 cup carrots
- 1 cup frozen corn
- 1 cup of water
- 1 cup cooked potatoes

- flour

- frozen peas

- seasonings (garlic, parsley, onion powder)

- milk

Start with your basic chicken soup recipe and add the following items to a pot: chicken (cooked,) chicken broth powder, seasonings, corn, carrots, cooked potatoes, peas, water, and some milk. Whisk in a little flour to thicken the soup. Or you can make this in a crock pot by adding everything into it, and turning it into a soup you'll like and love. Cook on low for a couple hours until the vegetables are soft.

<u>Chicken Noodle Soup</u>

Ingredients:

- chicken (1 cup)

- water

- 2 - 3 carrots diced or already frozen from a bag

- frozen Corn

- chicken broth powder

- seasonings (garlic, parsley, onion powder)

- celery stalks (2 or 3 diced)

Put a pot onto the stove, bring your water to a boil, add a cup of noodles to the pot and boil them, until they are cooked and soft. (See recommended time on the box for noodle type.) Then add a tablespoon of chicken broth powder to a one cup measuring cup, fill it up water, whisk, then stir it into the pot. Then add some carrots, parsley seasoning, garlic powder, onion powder, cooked chicken, corn and celery. Cook until vegetables the are soft.

<u>Sausage Alfredo Pasta Dish</u>

Ingredients:

- olive oil (one tablespoon)

- noodles (1 cup)

- sausage (Italian style sausage links)

- white sauce (1 jar any type)

- water

- seasonings (ideas include: garlic, parsley, oregano, italian seasoning, onion powder)

NOTE: Because we have sensitive tummies we need to learn what seasonings work best for us. Experiment with your seasonings!

Get a pot out and put on the stove, then add olive oil. Bring half a pot of water to a boil, add a cup of noodles to the pot and boil them, until they are cooked and soft. (See recommended time on the box for noodle type.) Drain noodles and return to pot.

Then to a 2nd pot, fill halfway with water. Add sausage links and bring to a boil to get the salt out of it.

Then once done, let them cool off. Dice the sausage into chunks, add to the pot with your noodles. Stir and then add your white alfredo sauce to the pot. Finally add your seasonings to taste and that's it, serve hot.

<u>Chicken Soup and Biscuits</u>

Ingredients:

- chicken (1 cup cut up)
- spinach (1 cup frozen)
- 3 cups water
- 2 cups milk (dairy free)
- flour
- garlic powder, oregano and onion powder
- biscuits (1 can refrigerator biscuits) – Prepare these as listed on the package.

Cook your chicken first, then once done, cook your spinach. To a large pot add the milk and water, some seasonings. Whisk in one tablespoon of flour, then add chicken and spinach. Bring to a boil then simmer to thicken. Serve with biscuits.

<u>Chicken Rice Soup</u>

Ingredients:

- 1 cup chicken (already cooked and cut up)
- 1/2 cup white rice
- 1 cup carrots (diced)
- 1 cup celery (diced)
- 1 cup corn (frozen)
- 5 cups chicken broth

Put the crock pot on low and add all of your ingredients. Alternatively, you can cook on the stove on low. It will taste very good.

Chapter 10

I hope you all enjoyed my book, and if you have any questions about what I eat and drink or just want to chat about your sickness, go to my personal website:

www.mils09.wixsite.com/website

It's easy to find, go to the search bar on your computer on the internet and type it in the web address. And once you are on my website there is a chat box at the bottom of the page. You can message me anytime!

I may not have all of the answers you seek or want but, I hope I helped you enough, and to inspire you as much as I can.

Like said before, keep believing yourself and you'll be ok and ask your doctor if you need more help in your life.

I hope and pray you guys will enjoy this book, as much as I enjoyed writing it for you.

Have a blessed day and keep fighting the gastroparesis because I'm fighting with you, right along your side, my friend.

I hope you enjoyed my personal cookbook, Have fun always!!

Your friend, Missy Gordon

The End